YOUR KNOWLEDGE HAS VALUE

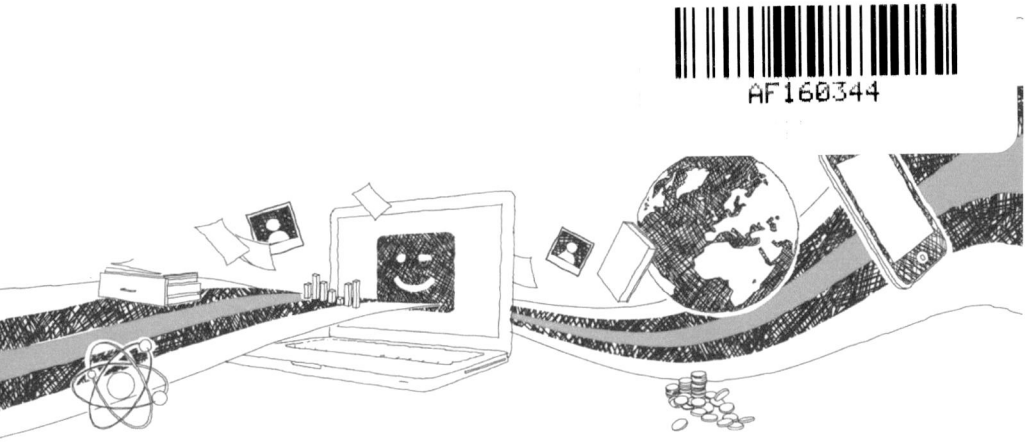

- We will publish your bachelor's and master's thesis, essays and papers

- Your own eBook and book - sold worldwide in all relevant shops

- Earn money with each sale

Upload your text at www.GRIN.com
and publish for free

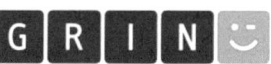

Bibliographic information published by the German National Library:

The German National Library lists this publication in the National Bibliography; detailed bibliographic data are available on the Internet at http://dnb.dnb.de .

This book is copyright material and must not be copied, reproduced, transferred, distributed, leased, licensed or publicly performed or used in any way except as specifically permitted in writing by the publishers, as allowed under the terms and conditions under which it was purchased or as strictly permitted by applicable copyright law. Any unauthorized distribution or use of this text may be a direct infringement of the author s and publisher s rights and those responsible may be liable in law accordingly.

Imprint:

Copyright © 2017 GRIN Verlag, Open Publishing GmbH
Print and binding: Books on Demand GmbH, Norderstedt Germany
ISBN: 9783668588547

This book at GRIN:

http://www.grin.com/en/e-book/381237/costs-and-benefits-of-the-international-flow-of-health-workers

Patrick Kimuyu

Costs and Benefits of the International Flow of Health Workers

GRIN Publishing

GRIN - Your knowledge has value

Since its foundation in 1998, GRIN has specialized in publishing academic texts by students, college teachers and other academics as e-book and printed book. The website www.grin.com is an ideal platform for presenting term papers, final papers, scientific essays, dissertations and specialist books.

Visit us on the internet:

http://www.grin.com/

http://www.facebook.com/grincom

http://www.twitter.com/grin_com

Costs and Benefits of the International Flow of Health Workers

Name: Patrick K. Kimuyu

Introduction 2
Drivers of Health Human Resources Migration 2
Costs and Benefits Dynamics Health Human Resources Migration 3
Welfare Costs of Health Human Resources Migration 6
Conclusion 7
References 9

Introduction

Health economics is seemingly becoming one of the most significant elements of healthcare sustainability. Despite the slowdown experienced in the realization of health transition in most countries, the current wave of globalization seems to have exerted a positive impact on global healthcare systems. However, shortages of health workers remain to be the greatest challenge to the development of healthcare systems, leading to imbalances in international human resources migration (Afzal et al., 2011). This challenge has also prompted many countries to adopt cost-effective healthcare reforms to improve the sustainability of healthcare systems and improve health outcomes. For instance, training for health workers has been intensifies in developing countries. OECD (2010) reports "Since 2000, the number of nursing graduates has increased at least by 50% in Australia, France, the United Kingdom and has doubled in Canada" (p. 4).

In 2008, Australia drafted primary healthcare reforms to ensure efficient flow of healthcare services by reducing healthcare expenditure. These reforms were designed based on the estimation of healthcare expenditure, which was expected to increase from 3.8 percent, in 2006-07 to 7.3 percent of the Gross Domestic Product, in 2046-47 (Commonwealth of Australia, 2009).

However, trends of healthcare costs are changing drastically, owing to the current international flow of healthcare professionals, which has influence health economics. Therefore, this paper will provide an overview on the costs and benefits of health human resources migration.

Drivers of Health Human Resources Migration

Economic reports indicate that cross-border flow of health professionals has been enhanced by globalization leading dramatic changes in low-income economies. The demand for health professionals in industrialized countries is influencing the flow of healthcare professionals from middle and low-income countries to developed countries such as the U.S, Australia and European countries. Currently, developed countries are experiencing enormous challenges in developing their healthcare systems because they lack adequate health human resources. Therefore, globalization seems to have enhanced the ability of developed countries by influencing the flow of healthcare professionals from other countries to fill the gap in their healthcare systems (Bundred, Martineau & Kitchiner, 2004).

Some of the principal drivers of health human resources migration, which have been created by globalization, include eased migration restrictions, health human resources policies, international financial support and economic situations in various regions.

Currently, the global labor market provides a significant platform for the exchange of professional skills, in which health professionals stream towards the region with high levels of employment opportunities. In regard to the flow of health human resources, deficits in high-income countries favor the migration of health professionals from low-income countries, owing to the eased migration restrictions. Ordinarily, health professionals who possess internationally accredited professional knowledge migrate abroad to seek for employment opportunities abroad, primarily in developed countries where deficits on health human resources are experienced because their professional knowledge is regarded to as a valuable commodity in the global job market (Bundred, Martineau & Kitchiner, 2004).

The second driver of health human resources migration is the deterioration of economic situations in various regions around the globe. For instance, inappropriately-timed market liberalization in Africa and Latin America has led to massive out-migration of health professionals leading to an unprecedented influx of nurses and doctors in the developed countries. Despite the continued efforts by the international monetary agencies to address market liberalization challenges in developing countries through the extension of grants and loans to the concerned countries, market stability remains a significant challenge, which is influencing migration of health professionals to high-income economies.

Costs and Benefits Dynamics Health Human Resources Migration

Ordinarily, international, macro and micro-economic dynamics influence the costs and benefits of health human resources migration. In regard to domestic macro-economic dynamics, there are several factors, which play a significant role in determining cross-border migrations. Some of these factors include economic growth rate, employment trends, and public expenditure on healthcare. On the other hand, economic, social and political stability has been found to influence the migration of health professionals. Moreover, judicial governance and political administrative policies influence health human resources flow in and out of the concerned country.

On the other hand, domestic micro-economic dynamics influence health human resources migration, more or less the same as macro-economic dynamics in a given country. For instance, structural and institutional features of the health sector influence the volume of migration streams of health professionals. In most cases, shortages of employment opportunities accompanied by poor compensation are believed to drive health workers to their country of choice in search of well-paying employment opportunities.

Moreover, global dynamics such as the mobility of medical human capital, changes in immigration policies and standardization of medical education influence cost and benefits of health human resources migration. For instance, developed countries experience an unprecedented demand and supply imbalances in their health labor markets, which favor migration of health workers from foreign countries (Forcier & Giuffrida, 2004).

Benefits of Health Human Resources Migration

From an economic perspective, cross-border migration of health workers is associated with several benefits, which make most countries allow foreigners to be integrated in their healthcare systems. Some of the most common benefits of health human resources migration include financial remittance flows, network externalities and social welfare.

In regard to financial remittance flows, source countries are believed to receive economic benefits from emigration of health human resources from their countries. For instance, the countries received foreign exchange from international revenue transfer, enabling them to sustain financial expenditures in their healthcare systems. According to the World Health Organization (2006), financial remittance flows involve millions of foreign currency, which are remitted to the source countries by migrants, and this has been observed to have reduced poverty in most developing countries (WHO, 2006). India is n outstanding example in regard to the contribution of financial remittance inflow from health emigrants.

India's Financial Remittance from Health Emigrants (Chishti, 2007)

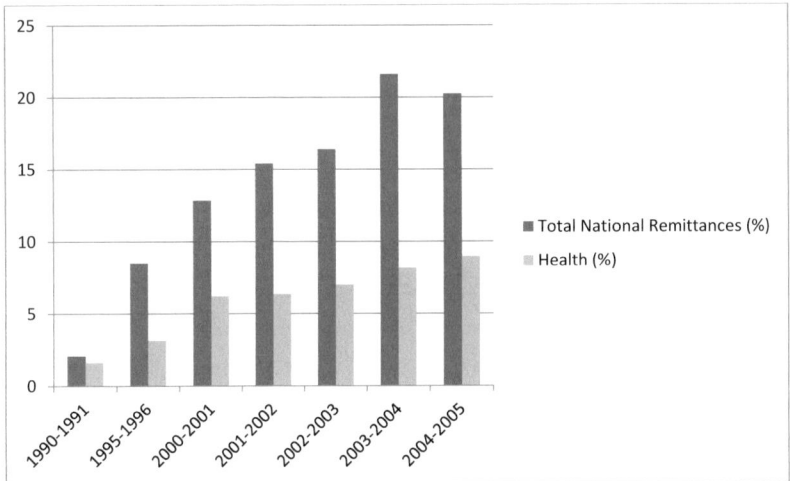

On the other hand, foreign revenue received from migrants helps to improve healthcare systems in developed countries by increasing budgetary allocation on health sector, and this leads to the improvement of public health in the source countries.

On the other hand, international migration of health workers contributes to network externalities in terms of trade, technology transfer and investment flows. Ordinarily, immigrants create extensive social and business networks, which enable developing countries to benefit from technology transfers. For instance, foreign direct investment by developed countries in developing countries facilitates the establishment of healthcare facilities in developing countries in the effort of harnessing business opportunities in these countries. As a result, foreign firms introduce foreign technology and advanced educational skills, which are integrated into the local health workforce leading to the improvement of healthcare systems (Wescott, 2006). Ideally, foreign direct investments are allowed by host countries so as to benefit from technological spill-over, which occur when foreign health firms release their employees after training them. Moreover, these foreign health firms provide employment opportunities to local health professionals enabling the host country to retain its health professionals because there are adequate employment opportunities.

Moreover, health human resources migration generates social benefits in health sectors of the involved countries. However, it is worth noting that the receiving countries are the ones who enjoy social benefits because international flow of health workers favors the migration of professionals from developing countries, where market environment is relatively unfavorable, to the developed countries such as the Unites States and European nations. Currently, most developing countries are experiencing an unprecedented medical brain drain while developed countries are harnessing these opportunities for social and economic gains. This issue has prompted developing countries to design numerous non-financial and financial health workers' retention policies to prevent extensive brain drain in their health sectors (Robinson, 2007).

On the other hand, international migration of health human resources benefits the host countries by filling the shortages with health professionals in their healthcare systems. For instance, the U.S, Australia and Canada have been relying on foreign health workers in their healthcare systems. These countries experience shortages of health professionals in the health sector; thus, prompting them to outsource health workers from developing countries to fill the gap (Global Health Watch, 2006). Packer et al (2008) report that at present, "all depend heavily on foreign-trained health professionals to cover important gaps in their HHR supply" (p. 217).

In contrast, "many health workers from the Philippines and Indonesia migrate to countries within SE Asia and to the rest of the world" (Houng et al. 2011, p. 776).

Welfare Costs of Health Human Resources Migration

In contrast, international migration of health human resources has been found to encompass numerous welfare costs. The first welfare cost of health human resources migration is the medical brain drain, in which the source country experiences enormous loss of health worker to foreign nations with improved employment environment (Docquier & Sekkat, 2006).

Ordinarily, medical brain drain leads to an unprecedented shortage of health professionals in the source country, primarily through occupation-specific human capital costs. For instance, emigration of health human resources causes loss of the most significant human capital assets.

Some of the human capital assets lost through health workers emigration include expertise of healthcare professionals, productive skills and experience. Surprisingly, most developing countries require a large health workforce because they are facing enormous healthcare challenges. However, their economies do not enable them to meet the required physician-patient ratio. It is reported that, the source country incurs a double loss because the loss of health professional who are educated and trained using the local economic resources.

Therefore, developing countries experience enormous human resource costs from the high rates of emigration of health workers, leading massive medical brain drain (Robinson, 2007).

On the other hand, emigration of health workers affects the economic growth of the source country. In most cases, source countries lose revenue, which could have been generated from employment income. In addition, these countries experience deficits in gross domestic product, leading to an unprecedented reduction of fiscal income.

Moreover, source countries incur enormous costs in replacing health workers who leave their employment opportunities in the local public health sector for employment in international health markets. On the other hand, significant losses are incurred owing to the lack of non-emergency care which leads to high mortality rates. In most cases, specialist care becomes scarce for patients.

In addition, host countries incur income losses arising from foreign tax revenues. These losses may lead to the reduction of the host country's gross domestic product; thus, influencing economic growth. Ordinarily, the reduction in gross domestic product of the host country causes an increase in the living standards of the local population.

It is also believed that international migration of health workers influences epidemiological transitions of the source countries. For instance, source countries experience constrains in medical research capacities, which are fundamental in reducing the burden of diseases. Surprisingly, developing countries have lagged behind with slow realization of epidemiological transitions, and yet they are incurring immense human resource costs through emigration of their health workforce. Currently, developing countries, primarily in the Sub-Saharan Africa the Caribbean Region are experiencing immense health challenges, which are caused by infectious diseases such as HIV/AIDS, tuberculosis and malaria (Hagopian et al., 2004). In addition, these countries are experiencing losses caused by in-migration, in which health workers are not absorbed into the national workforce, owing to economic challenges (Packer, Ronald & Runnels, 2008).

Conclusion

In a brief conclusion, international flow of health workers encompasses benefits and costs. This influences both local and global health economics, and it is believed to interfere with global health equity. Currently, international flow of health workers has increased significantly owing to the impact of globalization, which enables cross-border migrations.

Some of the benefits of health human resources migration include the generation of foreign income by the source countries, financial remittance flows and network externalities. Network externalities enhance technology transfer in healthcare systems. It also creates investment flows and open up new business opportunities for foreign investors in health sectors of developing countries.

However, international flow of health professionals cause welfare costs, primarily in the source countries owing to increased brain drain. As a result, some developing countries are designing healthcare reforms, which will enable them to restrict international mobility of health human resources while reducing wastage of in-country workforce (Gent & Skeldon, 2006).

References

Afzal, M. et al. (2011). The Global Health Workforce Alliance: Increasing the Momentum for Health Workforce Development. *Rev Peru Med Exp Salud Publica*, 28(2): 298-306. Retrieved from http://www.who.int/workforcealliance/media/photos/GHWA_Article_Jul2011.pdf

Bundred, P., Martineau, T., & Kitchiner, D. (2004). Factors affecting the global migration of health professionals. *Harvard Health Policy Review*, 5: 77–87.

Chishti, M. (2007). *The Rise in Remittances to India: A Closer Look*. Retrieved from http://www.migrationinformation.org/Feature/display.cfm?ID=577

Commonwealth of Australia (2009). *Primary Health Care Reform in Australia Report to Support Australia's First National Primary Health Care Strategy*. Retrieved from http://www.yourhealth.gov.au/internet/yourhealth/publishing.nsf/Content/nphc-draftreportsupp-toc/$FILE/NPHC-supp.pdf

Docquier, F. & Sekkat, K. (2006). *Brain Drain and Inequality across Nations*. Retrieved from http://dev3.cepr.org/meets/wkcn/4/4556/papers/docquier.pdf

Forcier, S. & Giuffrida, A. (2004) "Impact, Regulation and Health Policy Implications of Physician Migration in OECD Countries." *Human Resource for Health, 2(12)*.

Gent, S., & Skeldon, R. (2006). *Skilled Migration: Healthcare Policy Options*. Brighton, UK: Development Research Centre on Migration, Globalization and Policy. Retrieved from http://www.migrationdrc.org/publications/briefing_papers/BP6.pdf

Global Health Watch (2006). *Global Health Crisis*. Retrieved from http://www.ghwatch.org/2005_report_contents.php

Hagopian, A. et al. (2004). *The Migration of Physicians from Sub-Saharan Africa to the United States of America: Measures of the African Brain Drain*. Retrieved from http://www.human-resources-health.com/content/2/1/17

Huong, N. et al. (2011). Human Resources For Health In Southeast Asia: Shortages, Distributional Challenges, And International Trade In Health Services. *The Lancet*, 377: 769-780. Retrieved from http://indiaenvironmentportal.org.in/files/Health%20in%20Southeast%20Asia.pdf

OECD (2010). *International Migration of Health Workers: Improving International Co-Operation to Address the Global Health Workforce Crisis*. Retrieved from http://www.oecd.org/migration/mig/44783473.pdf

Packer, C., Ronald, L., & Runnels, V. (2008). *Globalization and the Cross-Border Flow of Health Workers*. Retrieved from http://www.globalhealthequity.ca/electronic%20library/Globalization%20and%20the%20Cross-Border%20Flow%20of%20Health%20Workers.pdf

Robinson, R. (2007). *The Costs and Benefits of Health Worker Migration from East and Southern Africa (ESA): A Literature Review*. Retrieved from http://www.nsi-ins.ca/wp-content/uploads/2012/10/2007-The-Costs-and-Benefits-of-Health-Worker-Migration-from-East-and-Southern-Africa-ESA-A-Literature-Review.pdf

Wescott, C. (2006). Harnessing Knowledge Exchange among Overseas Professionals. *International Public Management Review*, 7(1): 30-69.

WHO, (2006). *The World Health Report – Working Together for Health*. World Health Organization. Retrieved from http://www.who.int/whr/206/en

YOUR KNOWLEDGE HAS VALUE

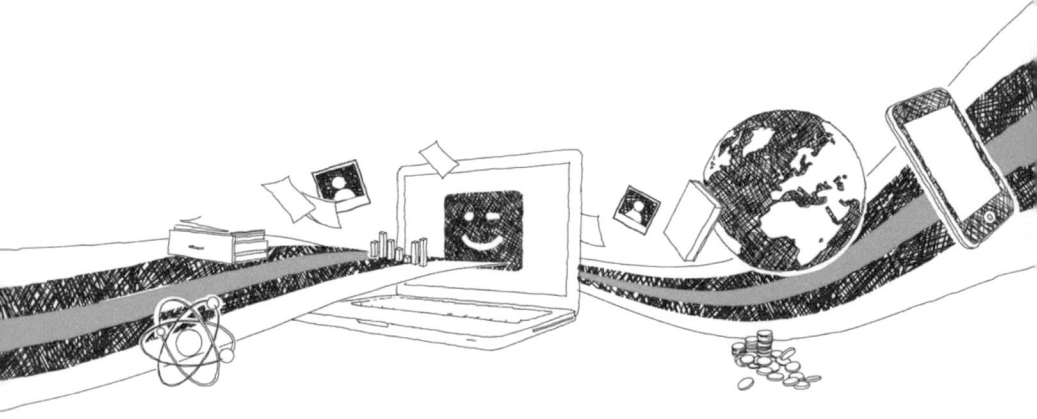

- We will publish your bachelor's and master's thesis, essays and papers

- Your own eBook and book - sold worldwide in all relevant shops

- Earn money with each sale

Upload your text at www.GRIN.com
and publish for free

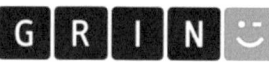